Breaking the Barriers:

Self-Managed Abortion Made Safe and Accessible!

Table of Contents

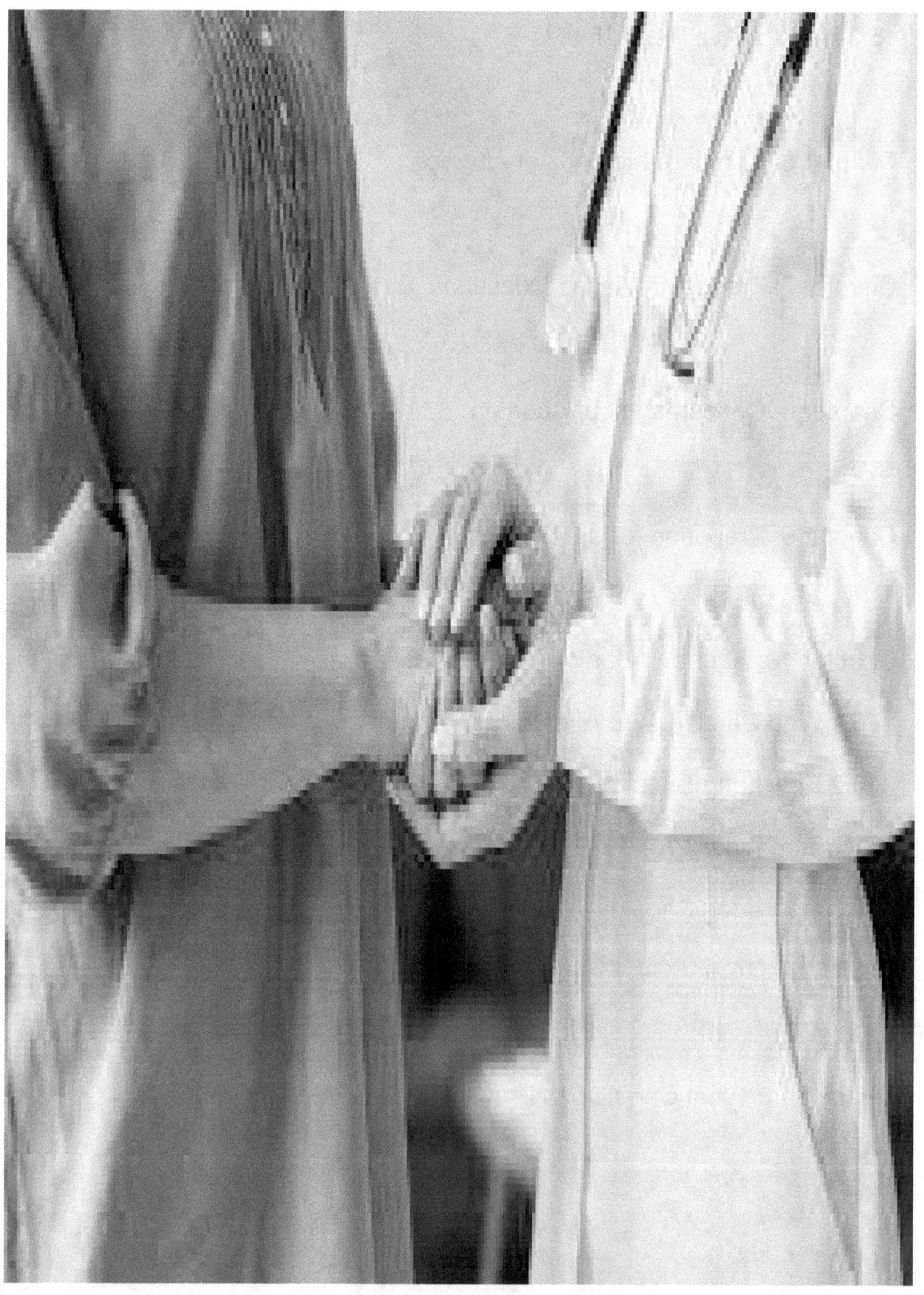

Introduction:

Breaking Barriers: Self-Directed Abortions Are Safe and Affordable *IF*... YOU HAVE THE RIGHT INFORMATION!

In many parts of the world, women face numerous barriers to accessing safe and legal abortion care. These barriers can range from limited health facilities and resources to restrictive laws that prevent women from exercising their reproductive rights. For women in such circumstances, self-abortion becomes an option worth considering. "Breaking the Barriers: Self-Managed Abortion Made Safe and Accessible" is a comprehensive guide designed to help women who find themselves in areas without easy access to medical facilities or where the law limits their ability to obtain abortion care.

This book is specifically tailored to the needs and concerns of women seeking self-directed abortion as a viable alternative. It provides a wealth of information, practical guidance and support to help women navigate this process safely, while emphasizing the importance of individual autonomy and informed decision-making. It serves as a beacon of hope for those who may feel trapped by the limitations of their circumstances.

This book is aimed at resilient women who, due to geographic, social or legal constraints, cannot seek professional medical help for their abortion-related needs. It aims to empower them by equipping them with the knowledge and resources necessary to make informed decisions about their reproductive health.

The chapters in this book cover a wide range of topics, starting with the early signs of pregnancy and the various methods of confirming it. From there, we delve into the specifics of self-induced abortion and explore safe and effective methods such as abortion with the pill, suction abortion, and dilation and evacuation (D&E). Each method is explained in detail with respect to safety aspects, instructions for proper use, management of pain and potential side effects, and how to assess abortion success.

Throughout the book, we put a lot of emphasis on safety and self-care. We provide detailed information on how to prevent and manage potential complications, recognize danger signs and seek appropriate medical attention if needed. In addition, we address common concerns and frequently asked questions, offering reassurance and practical advice to ease any worries.

We understand that abortion can be a sensitive and emotionally demanding process. That is why we devoted a chapter to post-abortion care, which deals with the physical and emotional well-being of individuals after the procedure. We discuss signs of recovery, prevention of infections, resumption of sexual activity and the possibility of effective contraception for the future.

"Breaking the Barriers: Self-Managed Abortion made safe and Accessible" is more than just a guide; is a testament to the tenacity, strength and determination of women who fight against oppressive systems. It recognizes their agency and their right to control their bodies and their future. By providing accurate, evidence-based information and practical guidance, we hope to empower women to make informed decisions about their reproductive health, despite the barriers they face.

We strongly believe that access to safe abortion care is a basic human right. Through this book, we strive to break down the barriers that prevent women from accessing quality healthcare and support their journey to self-determination. We hope that every woman who reads this book will find the information, courage, and support necessary to overcome challenges and regain control over her reproductive decisions.

Let's break down barriers together and empower women around the world to make safe and informed decisions about their bodies, lives and futures.

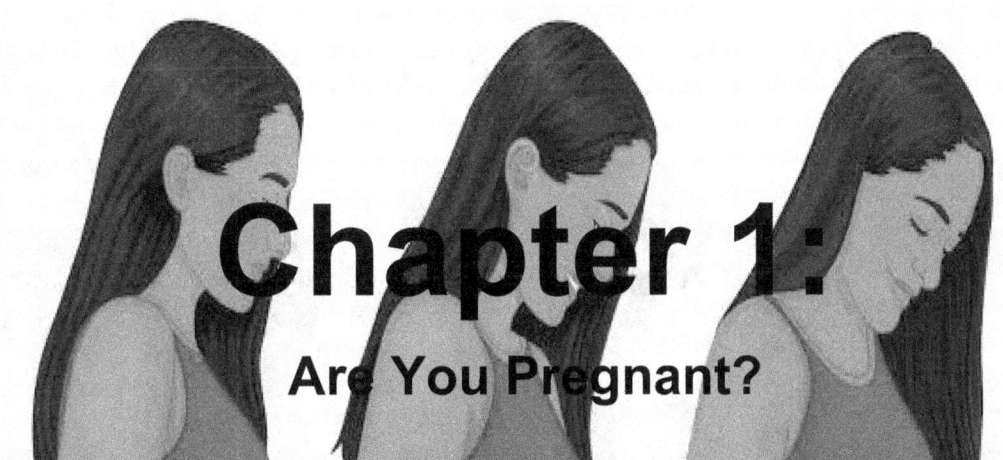

Chapter 1:

Are You Pregnant?

Discovering a potential pregnancy can be a pivotal moment in a woman's life. Whether it was planned or unexpected, the realization brings about a myriad of emotions, questions, and considerations. In this chapter, we will explore the various aspects of determining pregnancy and understanding the signs that may indicate its presence. We will also delve into the different methods of confirming pregnancy, providing you with the knowledge and tools to take control of your reproductive health.

If you think you are pregnant and do not want to be, this book can help you understand your options for ending the pregnancy without endangering your health. But first, make certain you are pregnant. After you are sure, use the pregnancy calculator to estimate for how long. Then you can find which are the safest methods for ending your pregnancy.

1.1 Signs of pregnancy

If pregnant, you may have some or all of these signs:
Monthly bleeding does not happen
Breasts feel sore and get bigger
Nausea or vomiting without being ill. Many pregnancies cause nausea in the morning (which is why it is called "morning sickness"), but some people feel slightly nauseous all day or never have nausea.
Need to pass urine more often
Tiredness

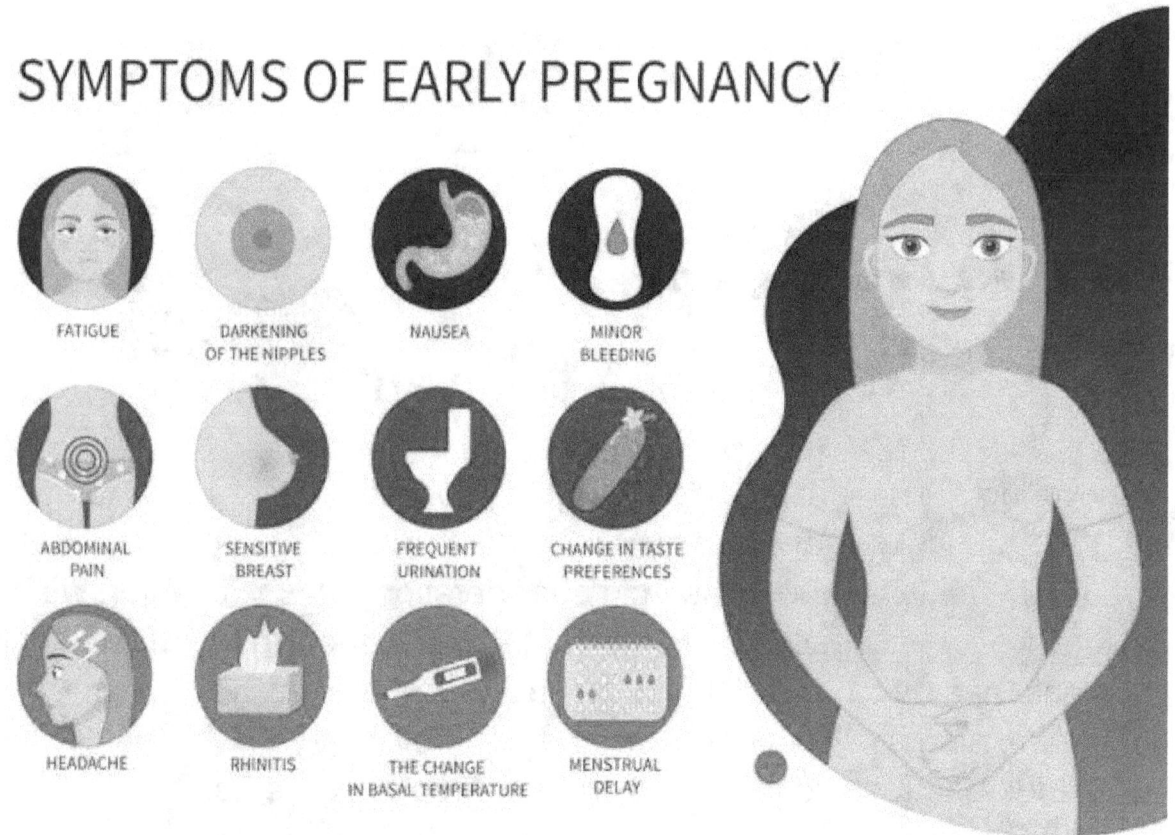

SYMPTOMS OF EARLY PREGNANCY

FATIGUE

DARKENING OF THE NIPPLES

NAUSEA

MINOR BLEEDING

ABDOMINAL PAIN

SENSITIVE BREAST

FREQUENT URINATION

CHANGE IN TASTE PREFERENCES

HEADACHE

RHINITIS

THE CHANGE IN BASAL TEMPERATURE

MENSTRUAL DELAY

A positive pregnancy test
Because some signs of pregnancy are also caused by other problems, a pregnancy test is the surest way to know if you are pregnant. Get a pregnancy home-testing kit that tests your urine.
This book can help a woman learn about how to end a pregnancy safely. Our "Safe Pregnancy and Happy Birth" handbook has useful information if you choose to continue with your pregnancy.

1.2 Pregnancy Test

A home pregnancy test using a urine PT strip is a convenient and commonly used method to detect pregnancy. These tests are designed to detect the presence of human chorionic gonadotropin (hCG), a hormone produced by the placenta during pregnancy, in a woman's urine.

Here are the steps to take a pregnancy test at home using a urine PT strip:

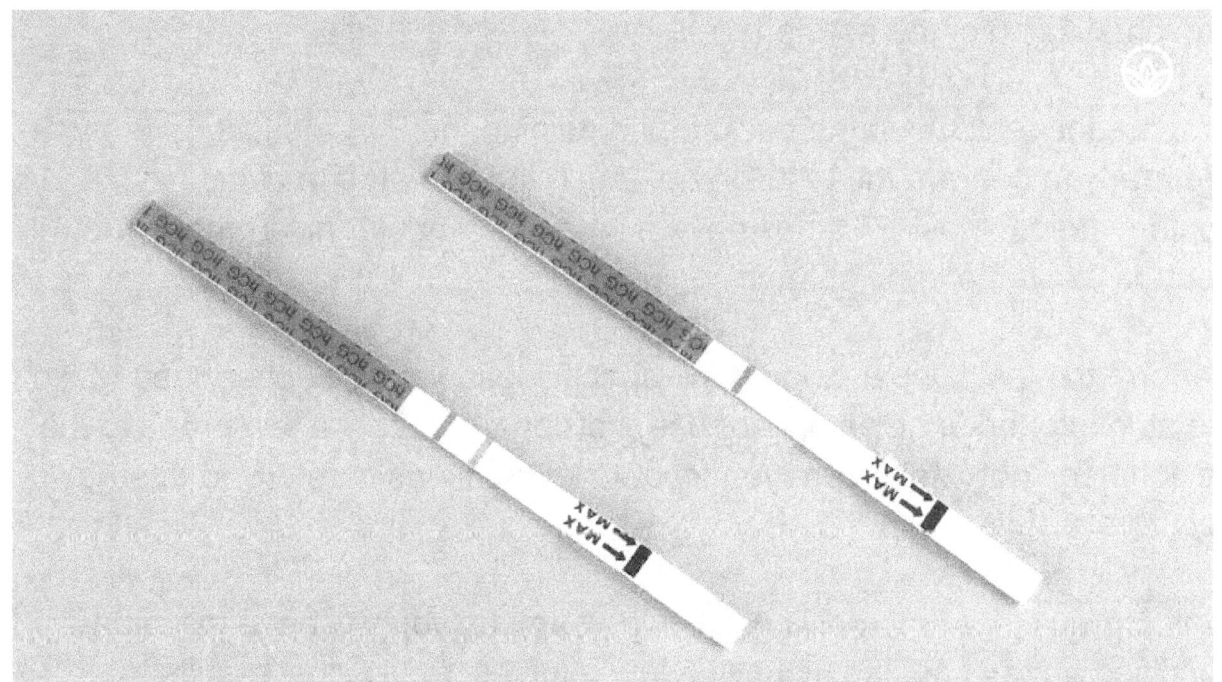

Choosing the right time: It is important to wait until you have missed your period before taking a pregnancy test. Taking the test too early can lead to a false-negative result, as hCG levels may not yet be detectable. Most tests recommend waiting at least a week after missing your period to get accurate results.

Buy a reliable urine PT strip: There are many brands available in the market and it is important to choose a reliable and reputable one. Look for a test that has a high sensitivity for hCG and provides clear instructions for its use.

Read the instructions carefully: Each brand may have slightly different instructions, so it is important to carefully read and understand the instructions that come with the test. Pay attention to the recommended test time and any specific instructions for accurate results.

Collect a urine sample: You will need to collect a urine sample for the test. It is generally recommended to use a first morning urine sample as it has higher concentrations of hCG. However, if you are testing later in the day, be sure to avoid excessive fluid intake for several hours before the test to prevent dilution of the hormone.

Prepare the test: Open the package containing the PT strip just before you are ready to perform the test. Do not touch the test strip to avoid contamination. Most PT strips have a small rectangular area where you will need to place the urine sample.

Perform the test: Depending on the specific test, you will either need to dip the strip into the urine sample or use a dropper to apply a few drops to the designated spot. Make sure you follow the directions carefully to ensure accurate results.

Wait for results: After applying the urine sample, you will have to wait a specified amount of time, usually a few minutes, for the test results to appear. It is important to follow the recommended waiting time, as reading results too soon or too late can lead to inaccurate interpretations.

Interpretation of Results: After the waiting period, carefully read and interpret the results according to the instructions provided. Most tests use lines or symbols to indicate whether the test is positive or negative. A control line should appear to confirm that the test is working correctly. The presence of a second line, even a weak one, usually means a positive result.

Follow up if necessary: If the test result is positive, it is recommended to schedule an appointment with a health care provider to confirm the pregnancy. They may perform additional tests, such as a blood test or ultrasound, to verify the results and provide appropriate prenatal care instructions.

Repeat the test if necessary: In some cases, if the initial test is negative, but you still have pregnancy symptoms or have not had your period, it may be recommended to repeat the test after a few days. This is because hCG levels may not be detectable early and may increase over time.

It is important to note that although home pregnancy tests are generally accurate, there may be cases of false negative or false positive results. Factors such as using an expired test, not following directions properly, or testing too soon can affect the reliability of the results. If you have any doubts or concerns, it is always best to consult your doctor.

Chapter 2:

Safe Methods of Abortion

To know which abortion method will be best for you, you need to know how many weeks you are pregnant. The earlier you are in pregnancy, the safer the abortion.

Abortion pills can be used for up to 20 weeks, but are safest during the first 10 weeks and can be done from home. After 10 weeks, it is safer if done in a clinic. From 10 to 14 weeks, a suction abortion is a better option. After 14 weeks, a D&E abortion is a better option.

2.1 Abortion with Pills

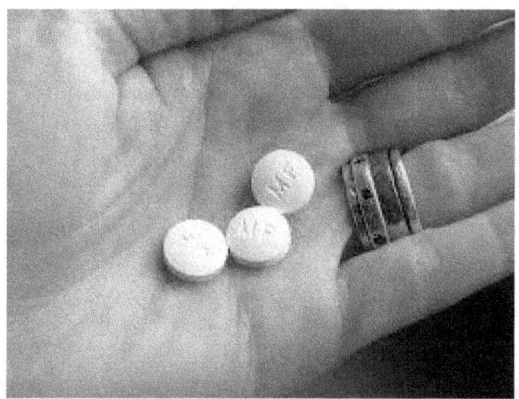

Two medications, misoprostol and mifepristone, can be used to safely terminate a pregnancy. Misoprostol can be taken alone, but abortions are most successful when taken together. Drug names can be easily confused; remember "misoprostol (misoprostALL) is the one to ALWAYS use".

Misoprostol causes your uterus to contract and push out the pregnancy. It's similar to having a miscarriage.

Mifepristone prevents your body from producing progesterone, which is needed to maintain a pregnancy, and softens your cervix so that pregnancy comes out easier.

Using medication to induce an abortion is called "medical abortion" or "abortion with the pill."

Misoprostol is a widely available drug also used to treat stomach ulcers or by midwives after childbirth. It is available in many countries with many different brands. It can be used alone to induce abortion, but is more effective when used in combination with mifepristone.

Mifepristone is a drug used only for abortion. It does not work by itself, only in combination with misoprostol. The most effective is the combined use of mifepristone and misoprostol. However, Mifepristone is not available in all countries.

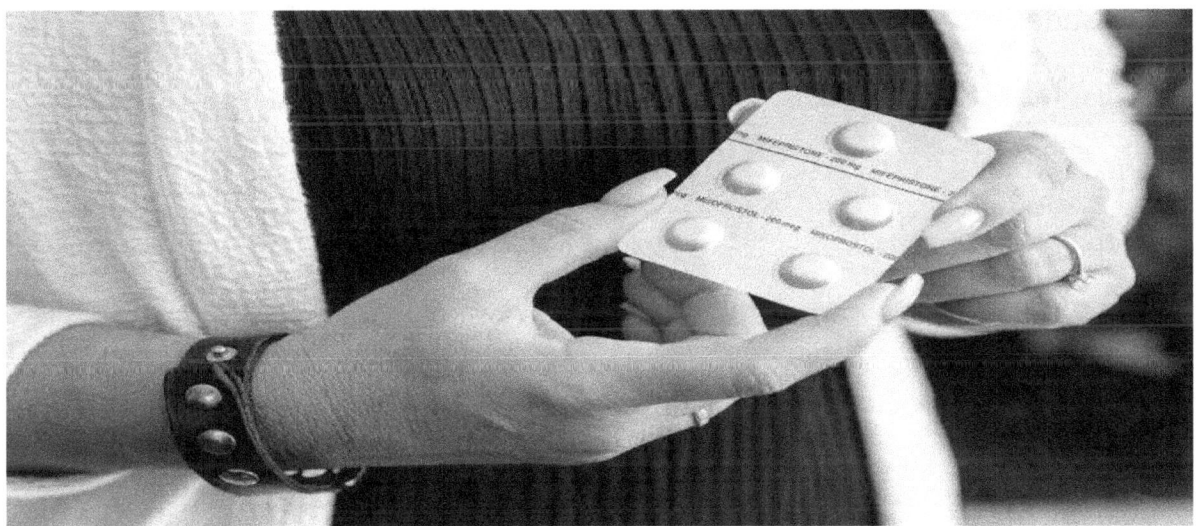

Misoprostol is found in many different countries under the following trade names:

- Asotec
- Chromalux
- Cyprostol
- Cyrus

- He felt

- Cytopan

- Cytotec

- Gastrula

- Isovent

- Contraction

- Noprostol

- Misoclear

- Misodel

- Misofar

- misoprolene

- Mixture

- misotrol

- Misoprostol

- Prostokos

- Vagiprost

Misoprostol also comes in a pill combined with diclofenac, an NSAID pain reliever, etc

even more brands.

2.1.1 How Safe is an Abortion with Pills?

With proper medication, abortion pills are very safe and effective, no matter how old you are. And because nothing is inserted into your uterus (womb), there is little risk of infection.

When to use abortion pills: Best before 10 weeks (70 days) of pregnancy, but can be used effectively for 20 weeks.

Where to get a pill abortion: During the first 10 weeks of pregnancy, you can get a pill abortion at home or at a clinic. If you have an abortion at home, it is best to have someone available to help you get to the clinic within an hour if you have very heavy bleeding or other problems.

After 10 weeks of pregnancy, there should be an abortion using pills at the clinic.

2.1.2 Who should not use abortion pills

- If you have had pain or bleeding during this pregnancy
- If you are more than 13 weeks pregnant and have had 2 previous cesarean deliveries (C-section).
- If you have any serious health problems such as:
  - heart disease
  - severe anemia
  - bleeding disorder
- chronic adrenal failure
- If you are taking blood thinners such as warfarin, dabigatran or rivaroxaban
- If you have ever had an allergic reaction to mifepristone or misoprostol
- If you are currently using an IUD (a small device inserted into the uterus to prevent pregnancy). After the IUD is removed, you can have an abortion using the pill.

Abortion pills will not end an ectopic pregnancy (tubal pregnancy). Symptoms include abdominal pain or bleeding.

2.1.2.1 Ectopic pregnancy

An ectopic pregnancy occurs when a fertilized egg implants outside the uterus, most commonly in the fallopian tube. This is a serious condition that requires immediate medical attention. Here are some signs and symptoms of an ectopic pregnancy:

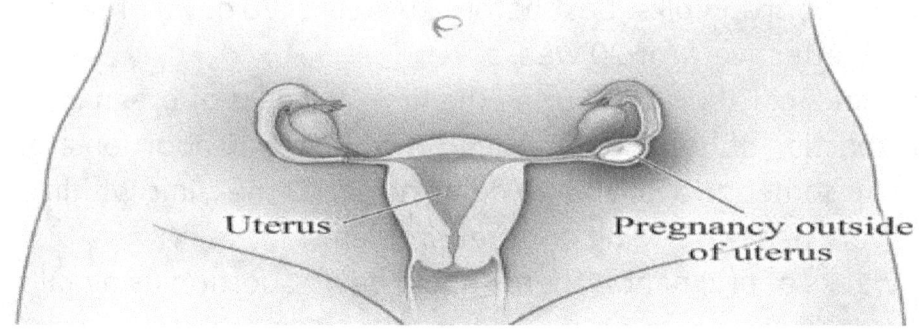

1. Abdominal or pelvic pain: This is one of the most common symptoms of an ectopic pregnancy. The pain is often sharp and can be localized to one side of the abdomen or pelvis. It may come and go or be persistent.

2. Vaginal Bleeding: There may be light vaginal bleeding or spotting that can be mistaken for a normal period. Bleeding may be lighter or heavier than usual and may be accompanied by pelvic pain.

3. Shoulder pain: In some cases, an ectopic pregnancy can cause irritation of the diaphragm, which can lead to pain in the shoulder area. This is known as "referred shoulder tip pain" and may be a sign of internal bleeding.

4. Weakness, dizziness or fainting: If an ectopic pregnancy ruptures and causes internal bleeding, it can lead to symptoms such as weakness, dizziness, lightheadedness or even fainting. This means a medical emergency and requires immediate care.

5. Gastrointestinal symptoms: Some women may experience symptoms similar to gastrointestinal problems such as nausea, vomiting, diarrhea or constipation. These symptoms can occur due to the effects of an ectopic pregnancy on the digestive system.

6. Missed periods or abnormal menstrual bleeding: In some cases, women with ectopic pregnancy may notice missed periods or irregular bleeding. However, it is important to note that these symptoms can also be associated with other conditions, so they are not just about an ectopic pregnancy.

It is important to remember that the symptoms of an ectopic pregnancy can vary from person to person and some women may not experience any symptoms until the condition worsens. If you suspect you may have an ectopic pregnancy or have any of the above symptoms, it is important to seek medical attention immediately. Early diagnosis and treatment are essential to prevent complications and ensure your well-being.

2.1.3 How to use abortion pills

There are 2 ways to take abortion pills.

Take misoprostol alone: Take the first dose of misoprostol. Painful cramping and heavy bleeding with clots can start as early as 30 minutes after taking misoprostol, although it can take up to 12 hours to start. Three hours after the first dose, take the next dose and 3 hours after that, take the last dose. You must take all 3 doses to complete the abortion, even if the cramping and heavy bleeding starts immediately after the first dose. Your bleeding will be heavier and last longer than a normal period – usually up to a week and often with continued spotting for 4 to 6 weeks until your period returns.

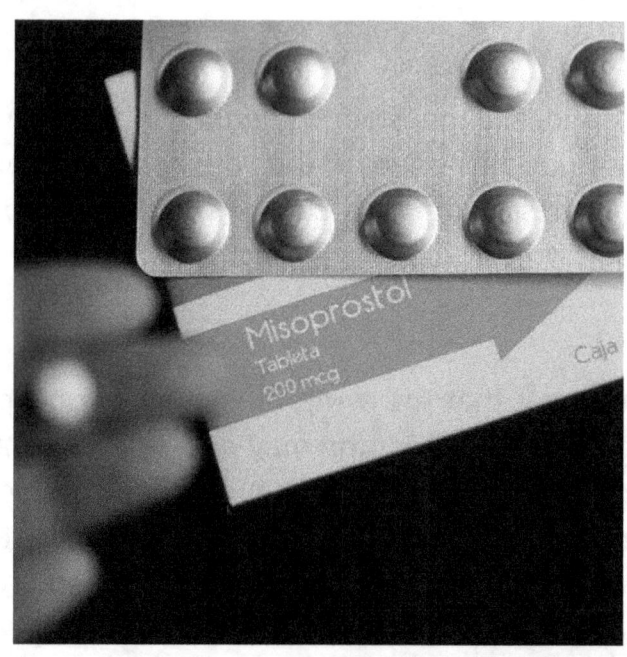

Use a combination of mifepristone and misoprostol: Take the mifepristone first. Most people feel nothing from taking this medicine, though you may have nausea or spotting. One to two days after taking the mifepristone, when it is convenient for you, take the misoprostol. But if your pregnancy is closer to 10 weeks, then wait to take the misoprostol closer to 48 hours. Within 2 hours of taking the misoprostol, and sometimes as soon as 30 minutes, you will feel strong cramping and bleeding will begin. Your bleeding will be heaviest, sometimes with clots, for 4 to 6 hours after taking the misoprostol. Then it will get lighter and last for about 2 weeks. Light bleeding and spotting may last up to 4 weeks.

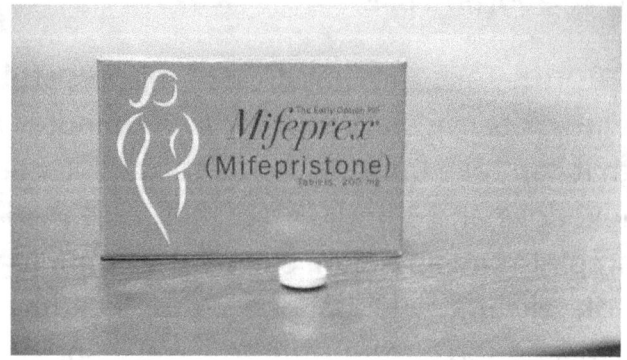

2.1.4 How long does it take?

Taking misoprostol alone: usually 7 to 8 hours after starting misoprostol, but sometimes the abortion takes up to 24 hours.

Using a combination of mifepristone and misoprostol: usually 4 to 6 hours after taking misoprostol, but longer for pregnancies longer than 13 weeks.

How long a miscarriage lasts varies from person to person because every body is different. It may take longer for someone who has never given birth before or those who are further along in their pregnancy. Bleeding and cramping may continue even after the abortion is complete.

2.1.5 How to manage pain during an abortion with pills

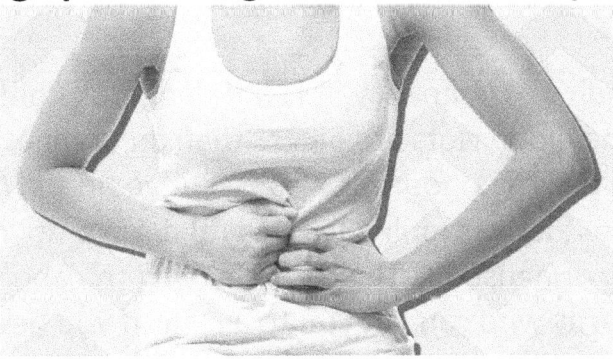

Not everyone has painful cramps during this type of abortion, but some women do. It helps to be prepared for this by having pain medicines on hand. It also helps to have a supportive friend or family member with you, to take you to a clinic if necessary and so you do not feel alone.

Cramping and pain should lessen a few hours after the abortion happens. To feel better, try:

- rest
- gentle massage
- use warm cloths, a hot water bottle, or a heating pad on your abdomen
- take ibuprofen or other NSAID pain medicines. Acetaminophen (paracetamol) will not help

- drink plenty of liquids
- ask a supportive friend or family member to spend time with you so you don't feel alone.

If your pain gets increasingly stronger, or if you are bleeding a lot, or if you have a high fever (38,5°C (101,4°F), <u>get help at a clinic or hospital</u>.

2.1.6 Normal bleeding and cramping

Bleeding and cramping (pain in the abdomen) are signs the abortion is happening. Cramping can be much like the pains of monthly bleeding, or it can be stronger or last longer.

Bleeding is part of ending a pregnancy. It is not dangerous unless it is very heavy. Get medical help if the blood clots are bigger than an orange, or if you soak through more than 2 pads in 1 hour for 2 consecutive hours. Also go to a clinic or hospital if you bleed without stopping for several days, or if you feel you might faint or are very dizzy or nauseous.. If you are having the abortion at home, plan to have someone nearby who can get you to a clinic if you need care.

2.1.7 How to use a combination of mifepristone and misoprostol
This is the best method for abortions up to 10 weeks. Using mifepristone and misoprostol together is effective 99% of the time.

There are 3 steps to a medical abortion using a combination of mifepristone and misoprostol.

Step 1: Swallow 200 mg of mifepristone with water.

Step 2: Wait 24 to 48 hours before taking misoprostol.

The more completely misoprostol dissolves in your mouth, as opposed to being swallowed, the less nausea it will cause. Using misoprostol in the vagina causes less nausea, but see the warning below about it not dissolving completely.

Step 3: Take 800 mcg (4 pills of 200 micrograms each) of misoprostol. When you let it dissolve slowly in your mouth, instead of swallowing it, it causes less nausea. There is even less nausea caused by letting it dissolve in the vagina, but it does not always dissolve completely. See the warning below.

There are 3 ways to take misoprostol:

1. Deep in the vagina

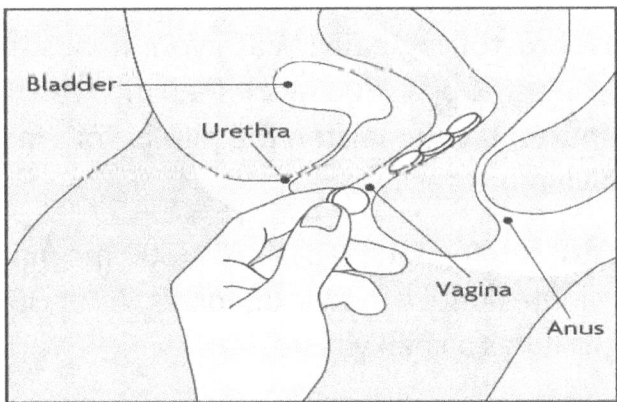

2. Under the tongue

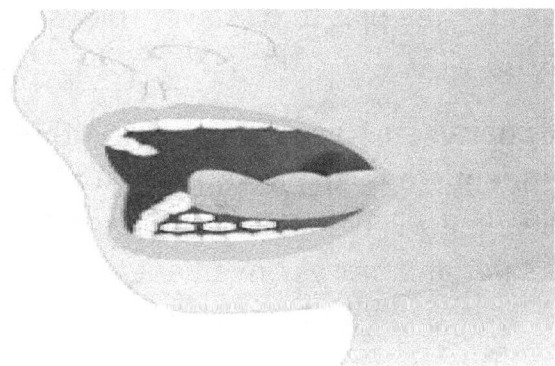

3. On each side of the mouth in between cheek and gum

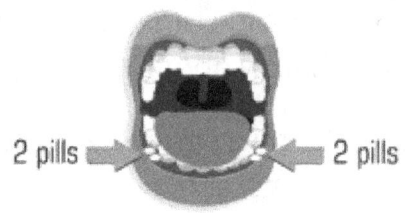

2 pills ➡ ⬅ 2 pills

IMPORTANT:

★ **For pregnancies longer than 9 weeks**, it is best to place misoprostol between the cheeks and gums (2 pills on each side).

  - **Using misoprostol vaginally:** Wash your hands thoroughly with soap and water. Push 4 pills (800 mcg) deep into the vagina and lie down for 30 minutes. If you moisten the pills before inserting them, they will dissolve more easily.

  - **Misoprostol sublingual:** Place 4 pills (800 mcg) under the tongue and wait 30 minutes until it slowly dissolves. After 30 minutes, swallow what's left. It has a chalky taste.

  - **Taking misoprostol between the cheeks and gums:** Place 2 pills (400 mcg) on each side of the mouth between the cheeks and gums. Wait 30 minutes for the pills to dissolve. Then swallow what's left. It has a chalky taste.

★ **For pregnancies between 10 and 13 weeks:** Although suction abortion is a better option, mifepristone and misoprostol can be used to terminate these pregnancies. Bleeding will be heavier and more severe pain and nausea may occur. It is safer and more convenient to do it in a clinic or medical facility.

★ **For pregnancies between 14 and 20 weeks:** Although a D&E abortion is the better option, mifepristone and misoprostol can still be used to terminate these pregnancies. Multiple and different doses are required and should be taken in a clinic or medical facility where it is safer and a trained provider can deal with any complications that may arise.

At the clinic, you will take 400 mcg (2 pills) every 3 hours until the abortion is complete, which can take up to 48 hours. Since the uterus is more sensitive to the drug after 13 weeks, it is important to avoid dangerous overdose and damage to the uterus, so take only 2 pills every 3 hours. Bleeding will be heavier, the miscarriage will take longer, and there may be more severe pain and nausea.

Also, if your abortion is not performed in a clinic, have a plan for disposing of the expelled blood and tissue. The tissue will be about 9 cm (3 ½ inches) long or larger and may have discernible parts. If you decide to bury it, make sure it's in a place where it won't be disturbed by people or animals.

WARNING: Where abortion is restricted, a woman can get into serious legal trouble if someone suspects that she attempted an abortion.

Since misoprostol usually does not dissolve completely in the vagina, undissolved pieces of pills may be found in the vagina in the event of a miscarriage and medical attention is needed. Taking misoprostol between the cheeks and gums or under the tongue is safer where abortion is illegal.

If you take mifepristone and do not take misoprostol for any reason, the pregnancy can continue without problems. However, it is also possible that mifepristone may cause an incomplete miscarriage and you may need to empty your uterus (womb) by suction.

Side effects

Abortion with pills can cause

- mild fever, below 38.5°C (101.4°F)
- nausea
- vomiting
- diarrhea

These side effects are less severe the longer you let misoprostol pills dissolve in your mouth rather than swallowing them.

Some people say these side effects feel like you have the flu. They are usually short-lived and go away on their own.

If you are breast-feeding, misoprostol may cause diarrhea in your baby. To reduce this risk, breastfeed right before taking the pills and then wait 4 to 5 hours before breastfeeding again. During this time, give the child a rehydration drink.

2.1.8 Taking misoprostol alone

The pill is the best method for abortion before 10 weeks. Taking misoprostol alone (without mifepristone) is effective in 85% of cases.

Each dose of misoprostol is 800 mcg. Three doses are needed 3 hours apart. So the total amount of misoprostol needed is 2400 mcg.

Usually there are 12 tablets of 200 mcg and each dose is 4 tablets.

Remember this by thinking 4-3-3: take 4 pills every 3 hours, 3 times.

(Recall) There are 3 ways to take misoprostol:

1. Deep in the vagina

2. Under the tongue

3. On each side of the mouth between the cheek and gums

IMPORTANT: For pregnancies longer than 9 weeks, it is best to take misoprostol between the cheeks and gums (2 pills on each side).

Step 1: Take 800 mcg (micrograms) of misoprostol. This is usually 4 tablets of 200 mcg each.

The more completely misoprostol dissolves in the mouth, as opposed to swallowing, the less nausea it will cause. Using misoprostol in the vagina causes less nausea, but see the warning below that it does not dissolve completely.

- **Using misoprostol vaginally:** Wash your hands thoroughly with soap and water. Push 4 pills (800 mcg) deep into the vagina and lie down for 30 minutes. If you moisten the pills before inserting them, they will dissolve more easily.

- **Misoprostol sublingual**: Place 4 pills (800 mcg) under the tongue and wait 30 minutes until it slowly dissolves. After 30 minutes, swallow what's left. It has a chalky taste.

- **Taking misoprostol between the cheeks and gums**: Place 2 pills (400 mcg) on each side of the mouth between the cheeks and gums, for a total of 4 pills (800 mcg). Wait 30 minutes for the pills to dissolve. Then swallow what's left. It has a chalky taste.

Step 2: Repeat in 3 hours and a final time 3 hours after that for a total of 3 doses (2,400 mcg total). It is important to take the second and third doses of misoprostol even if the bleeding has started and you think the miscarriage has already occurred. Taking all 3 doses will complete the abortion. If not, you will need medical attention.

- **For pregnancies between 10 and 13 weeks**: Although aspiration abortion is the better option, misoprostol (4 pills = 800 mcg every 3 hours, 3 times) can be used to terminate these pregnancies. Bleeding will be heavier and more severe pain and nausea may occur. It is safer and more convenient to do it in a clinic or medical facility.

- **For pregnancies between 14 and 20 weeks:** Although a D&E abortion is the better option, misoprostol can be used to terminate these pregnancies. Different doses are required and should be taken in a clinic or medical facility where it is safer and a trained provider can deal with any complications that may arise.

At the clinic, you will take 400 mcg (2 pills) every 3 hours until the abortion is complete, which can take up to 48 hours. Since the uterus is more sensitive to the drug after 13 weeks, it is important to avoid dangerous overdose and damage to the uterus, so take only 2 pills every 3 hours. Bleeding will be heavier, the miscarriage will take longer, and there may be more severe pain and nausea.

Also, if your abortion is not performed in a clinic, have a plan for disposing of the expelled blood and tissue. The tissue will be about 9 cm (3 ½ inches) long or larger and may have discernible parts. If you decide to bury it, make sure it's in a place where it won't be disturbed by people or animals.

WARNING: Where abortion is restricted, a woman can get into serious legal trouble if someone suspects that she attempted an abortion.

Since misoprostol usually does not dissolve completely in the vagina, undissolved pieces of pills may be found in the vagina in the event of a miscarriage and medical attention is needed. Taking misoprostol between the cheeks and gums or under the tongue is safer where abortion is illegal.

2.1.9 Adverse effects

Abortion with pills can cause

- mild fever, below 38.5C (101.4F)

- nausea

- vomiting

- diarrhea

These side effects are less severe the longer you let misoprostol pills dissolve in your mouth rather than swallowing them.

Some people say these side effects feel like you have the flu. They are usually short-lived and go away on their own.

If you are breast-feeding, misoprostol may cause diarrhea in your baby. To reduce this risk, breastfeed right before taking the pills and then wait 4 to 5 hours before breastfeeding again. During this time, give the child a rehydration drink.

2.1.10 How to find out if the abortion was successful

Even at 10 weeks, the pregnancy is only about an inch long, so it can be difficult to tell from what your body is shedding that the pregnancy is over after a pill abortion.

However, if the abortion was successful, the signs of pregnancy will disappear - morning sickness usually subsides within 24 hours, and your breasts will stop hurting in a few days. If the nausea lasts more than 2 days or if there is little or no bleeding after taking misoprostol, the abortion probably did not work.

If you are concerned that you have not had a successful abortion, go to a clinic or hospital where they will check you with an ultrasound (sonogram). If you're worried about legal issues, you can say you're worried about a miscarriage because you've had symptoms like bleeding, cramping, and pain in your lower back or abdomen.

Home pregnancy tests will not tell you if the abortion was successful. The hormones caused by the pregnancy remain in your body for about 3 weeks after the abortion, so the pregnancy test will be positive even if the abortion was successful.

2.1.11 Dangerous symptoms after abortion with pills

- Heavy Bleeding (Hemorrhage): Heavy bleeding seeps through more than 2 pads in 1 hour for 2 hours. Heavy bleeding is even more dangerous if you also feel dizzy or faint. Seek medical attention immediately for heavy bleeding.

- Large clots: The passage of blood clots that are larger than an orange is also a danger sign.

- Heavy bleeding and large clots are signs that the abortion may not have been successful. You should go to the clinic for a check-up, have an ultrasound done, and if the abortion was not successful, the clinic worker will empty your uterus (womb) by suction.

- Bleeding and cramping from a pill abortion is very similar to a miscarriage and is treated the same way. Doctors may not be able to tell the difference unless they find undissolved pieces of pills in your vagina.

- Fever: Fever is a sign of infection. Infection is more likely after a suction or D&E abortion, or if the abortion is incomplete.

  - If you have a fever after any type of abortion, you should seek medical attention, especially if:

  - fever is above 38.5°C (101.4°F) and lasts for more than 4 hours

  - fever is 38°C (100.4°F) and lasts more than 24 hours

  - you have fever and chills

- No bleeding: If you don't bleed after a pill abortion, the pills probably didn't work. You should go to the clinic to get more help.

2.1.12 Pills and vomiting

Medicines in abortion pills can make you sick. If you throw up the pills before the medicine dissolves and enters your body, there's a chance you won't get enough for the abortion to work. Here's what to do if this happens.

2.1.12 If you vomit misoprostol

If you vomit 30 minutes or more after taking misoprostol, the medicine will still be working. If you vomit before the 30 minutes are up, then the medicine may not be working and you should take it again, or moisten it and place it in your vagina instead of dissolving it in your mouth. If you live in an area where abortion with the pill can cause legal problems, remember that misoprostol can take a long time to completely dissolve in the vagina. If you need help later and are examined, pieces of pills may be found. If you are afraid of this, take the pills by letting them dissolve in your mouth.

2.1.14 If you vomit mifepristone

If you vomit 90 minutes or more after taking mifepristone, the medicine will still be working. But even if it's less than 90 minutes, if you take misoprostol as directed, the abortion will still work and you don't need to take another dose of mifepristone.

2.1.15 Nausea Control

Medicines may make you feel slightly nauseous. Try one of these:

Ondansetron: take 8 mg by mouth or rectally every 8 to 12 hours as needed.

Metoclopramide: take 20 mg by mouth, 1 time per day if needed. Do not use with alcohol.

Promethazine (Phenergan): take 25 mg by mouth, every 4 to 6 hours as needed.

Diphenhydramine (Benadryl): take 50 mg by mouth, every 6 to 8 hours as needed.

2.2 Abortion by suction

Aspiration abortion is a safe and effective method of abortion up to the 16th week of pregnancy. A trained provider uses suction to remove the pregnancy from the uterus (womb) using a plastic tube called a cannula. Suction is created either with a manual syringe (MVA) or an electric pump (EVA).

An MVA or EVA only takes about 5 to 10 minutes. It is usually done at a clinic, health station or doctor's office. Although safe up to 16 weeks, after 14 weeks a D&E abortion is recommended instead.

2.2.1 How safe is suction abortion?

Aspiration abortion, performed by a trained and experienced healthcare professional using sterile equipment and sterile technique, is a safe method of abortion up to 16 weeks. This method inserts a plastic tube through the cervix so the pregnancy can be removed by suction from the uterus. It is very important that the provider uses a sterile tube. Compared to a D&E abortion, suction abortions have a lower risk of infection, heavy bleeding, or bleeding or injury to the uterus or cervix.

Suctioning is safe and successful in almost all cases, both in abortion and in the treatment of incomplete or spontaneous abortion. Unsafe suction abortions, performed by unethical or untrained providers working in unsanitary conditions, usually only occur where abortion is restricted. Unsafe suction abortions can lead to medical emergencies such as infections and heavy bleeding.

When: This method can be used to terminate a pregnancy up to 16 weeks.

Where: Suction interruption should be performed **by a trained person** in the clinic.

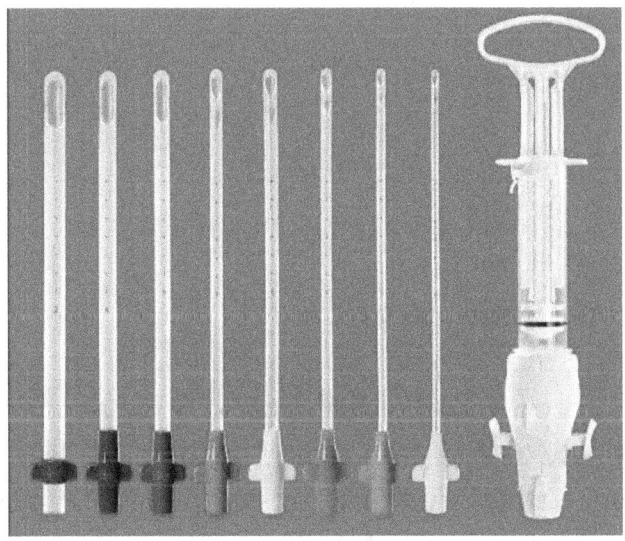

2.2.2 Who should not get an abortion by suction

Suction abortion is safe for anyone between 6 and 16 weeks pregnant.
Suction abortion does not end an ectopic pregnancy (tubal pregnancy).
Symptoms of an ectopic pregnancy include abdominal pain or bleeding.

What happened?

A suction abortion begins as a pelvic exam.
Your provider will ask you to lie down on the exam table and place your feet in stirrups. If you have a disability that makes it difficult for you to keep your legs apart, it may be easier for you if pillows or a person can comfortably support your legs in a position you can hold without straining your muscles.
The healthcare professional will gently open your vagina using a speculum. They then place a plastic tube called a cannula into the vagina and through the cervix into the uterus. If available, a healthcare professional may use a medicine such as lidocaine to numb the cervix so the procedure hurts less.

The healthcare professional then connects the cannula to either a manual syringe or an electric aspirator. Suction from either of these devices will pull the pregnancy out through the cannula. This takes about 10 minutes. During sucking, you will feel strong cramps and pressure in your abdomen.

After a miscarriage, your cramps will ease. If you take medicines such as ibuprofen, naproxen or acetaminophen (paracetamol), your pain should subside. You may be given medicines to prevent infection, such as doxycycline, azithromycin or metronidazole.

2.2.3 Medicine to prevent infection

An hour before the suction abortion, the provider may administer an antibiotic to prevent the possibility of infection after the abortion. Be sure to tell your provider if you've ever had an allergic reaction to medications.

You may be given one dose of one of these medicines to take by mouth:

Doxycycline: 200 mg (avoid doxycycline if breast-feeding); OR

metronidazole: 500 mg; OR

Azithromycin: 1 g.

2.2.4 Medicine to relieve pain

Pain medications can help relieve the pain of a suction abortion.

Ibuprofen: take 400 mg by mouth every 4 to 6 hours as needed. However, do not take more than 1200 mg in 24 hours.

Naproxen: Take 550 mg by mouth and take 275 mg every 6 to 8 hours thereafter. If necessary. Do not take more than 1375 mg in 24 hours.

Acetaminophen (paracetamol): take 1000 mg by mouth every 6 hours as needed. Do not take more than 4000 mg in 24 hours.

2.2.5 Bleeding and convulsions

You may have cramping or pain for a day after the abortion, as well as vaginal bleeding. But after the first day it shouldn't be more than light monthly bleeding and it should stop within 2 weeks.

2.2.6 How to find out if the abortion was successful

After a suction abortion, the provider looks at everything removed from the uterus to make sure the pregnancy has been completely removed. Morning sickness should disappear within a day; your breasts may hurt a little longer.

2.3 Dilation and Evacuation (D&E)

Dilation and Evacuation (D&E) is a safe and effective method of removing a pregnancy using a combination of suction and medical instruments. Medicines are often used to soften and open the cervix before a D&E.
D&E is usually used for pregnancies that are longer than 14 weeks. It may also be used to treat miscarriage to ensure that the entire pregnancy is removed from the uterus (womb).

2.3.1 How safe is D&E abortion?

A D&E abortion, performed by a trained and experienced healthcare professional using sterile equipment and sterile technique, is a safe method of abortion after 14 weeks to 24 weeks.
This method softens and opens (dilates) the cervix so that suction tubes and instruments can remove the pregnancy from the uterus. This is why it is very important that the provider uses sterile equipment to prevent infection.

Compared to suction or medical abortions, D&E abortions have a higher risk of infection, heavy bleeding, or bleeding or injury to the uterus or cervix.

Unsafe D&E abortions performed by unethical or untrained providers working in unsanitary conditions usually only happen where abortion is restricted. Unsafe D&E abortions can lead to life-threatening medical conditions such as heavy bleeding and serious infections.

When: This method can be used to terminate a pregnancy up to 24 weeks. It is a safe method after 14 weeks.

Where: A D&E should only be performed by a trained healthcare professional in a clinic or hospital with sterile conditions and equipment.

2.3.2 Who should not undergo a D&E abortion

A D&E abortion is safe for anyone at any age.

But a D&E abortion does not end an ectopic pregnancy (a pregnancy in the tubes). Symptoms of an ectopic pregnancy include abdominal pain and bleeding.

2.3.3 What happens?

First, a trained healthcare provider will gently open (dilate) your cervix using one of these methods:

- drugs (misoprostol or mifepristone, the same drugs used for abortion pills) given hours or days before the abortion;
- thin, absorbent rods called osmotic dilators are inserted into the cervix, where they absorb fluid and slowly expand over hours or days to open the cervix;
- mechanical dilation using instruments at the time of abortion.

Which method or combination of methods is used depends on how far along the pregnancy is, what resources are available at the clinic, and the health care provider's judgment.

You will be given antibiotics to protect against infection and some form of anesthesia to ease the pain. This usually means IV medication or sedation. Which drugs are used for pain management and anesthesia depends on how far along the pregnancy is, what resources are available at the clinic, your preferences, and the judgment of the health care provider.

After that, the health worker starts emptying the uterus. If dilators were used, they will be removed first and the provider will use suction and, if necessary, a grasping tool called forceps to remove the pregnancy. If you're awake, you'll feel strong pulls and cramps as your uterus empties.

Be sure to tell your healthcare provider if you are taking medications such as muscle relaxants or narcotics to avoid an overdose of pain relievers. If you have a disability that makes it difficult for you to keep your legs apart, it may be easier if pillows or a person can support your legs in a comfortable position that you can hold without straining your muscles.

2.3.4 How long does it take?

Dilation of the cervix using drugs or dilators usually takes a few hours if you are less than 18 weeks pregnant, and 1 or 2 days if your pregnancy is longer.

Once the cervix has opened sufficiently, the procedure itself takes about 20 minutes, but it depends on how far along the pregnancy is.

2.3.5 Medicine to prevent infection

An hour before the D&E abortion, the provider may administer an antibiotic to prevent the possibility of post-abortion infection. Be sure to tell your provider if you've ever had an allergic reaction to medications.

You may be given one dose of one of these medicines to take by mouth:

Doxycycline: 200 mg (avoid doxycycline if breast-feeding); OR

metronidazole: 500 mg; OR

Azithromycin: 1 g.

2.3.6 Medicine to relieve pain

Usually, the health care provider will give you an anesthetic such as lidocaine to relieve pain in the cervix. You may also be given strong IV drugs for pain or sleep. Which drugs are used to treat pain and anesthesia depends on the length of the pregnancy, the resources available at the clinic, your preferences, and the health care provider's judgment. Be sure to tell the health care provider if you are taking medications such as muscle relaxants or narcotics to avoid an overdose of pain relievers.

A pain reliever such as ibuprofen can help relieve the pain of a D&E abortion, but stronger pain relievers may be desired.

For ibuprofen, take 400 mg by mouth every 4 to 6 hours as needed. However, do not take more than 1200 mg in 24 hours.

Naproxen: Take 550 mg by mouth and take 275 mg every 6 to 8 hours thereafter. If necessary. Do not take more than 1375 mg in 24 hours.

Acetaminophen (paracetamol): take 1000 mg by mouth every 6 hours as needed. Do not take more than 4000 mg in 24 hours.

2.3.7 Bleeding and convulsions

It is normal to bleed a little right after a D&E abortion or to pass small clots. After that, the red bleeding stops for a few days or reduces to a light or moderate flow, turns pink or brown, can stop and start, but stops completely within 2 weeks.

Cramps usually subside within the first hour after the abortion.

2.3.8 After abortion

After a miscarriage, it takes time for your body to get back to normal. First the signs of pregnancy will disappear, then the bleeding or spotting will ease with the return of menstruation and it will be safe to resume sex. If you don't want to get pregnant, start using a birth control method right away.

If bleeding continues and you have pain or a fever above 101.4°F (38.5°C), see a doctor.

Search terms: after, after abortion, pain, fever, sore breasts, tender breasts, cramps, nausea, morning sickness, bleeding, spotting, infection, infection prevention, sex, sex recovery, birth control, contraception, family planning

Chapter 3:
Feeling Better

If you miscarried on the pill: Most people feel much better the day after taking misoprostol. You can usually return to your regular routines within a few days after the abortion.

If you have had a suction or D&E abortion: Cramps usually subside half an hour after the procedure. You can usually return to your regular routine within a few hours or a day after the abortion.

3.1 Symptoms of pregnancy disappear

If you have miscarried on the pill: Nausea usually goes away within 24 hours, but breast tenderness may persist for 1 or 2 weeks.

If you had a suction or D&E abortion: All symptoms, including nausea and sore breasts, should go away within a day.

If the signs of pregnancy, such as nausea and sore breasts, do not go away, you may still be pregnant, either in the uterus (womb) or in the tube (ectopic pregnancy). Home pregnancy tests will not be accurate soon after the abortion pill. Hormones caused by pregnancy last about 3 weeks in the body and will make the pregnancy test positive even if the abortion was successful. If you need confirmation that the abortion worked, get an ultrasound at the clinic.

If you have growing pains, you may have an ectopic pregnancy. This is an emergency. If you still have signs of pregnancy after 1 to 2 weeks, go to a clinic or hospital.

3.2 Bleeding

If you miscarried with pills: Bleeding will decrease after a few days. Light bleeding or spotting may continue until the next period.

If you have had a suction or D&E abortion: Vaginal bleeding may continue for up to 2 weeks. After the first day, it's usually like a light period, but you may have a few small clots.

3.3 Prevention of Infection

Wait at least 5 days after the abortion and 2 days after the bleeding has stopped before having sex or inserting anything into the vagina.

Especially if the cervix was opened for abortion, there is a greater chance of infection. If you have been given medications to take after a suction or D&E abortion, follow the directions and remember to take them all!

3.4 Start a contraceptive method

You can start using birth control (contraception) immediately after the abortion. If you do not protect yourself, you can get pregnant a few days after the abortion, before the next monthly bleeding. Start with a method to prevent pregnancy, such as:

A barrier method, such as condoms or a diaphragm, immediately after an abortion.

A hormonal method such as birth control pills, injections or implants on the same day as the abortion. If you start a hormonal method within 7 days of a miscarriage, it will prevent pregnancy. But if you wait more than 7 days to start, use a condom for a week, because hormones take time to provide full protection.

IUD. You can have an IUD inserted as soon as you are sure that the abortion was successful and there was no infection, about 3 days after the abortion. Use a condom until the IUD is in place.

If you are very sure that you never want to get pregnant again, you can have an operation (called a "tubal ligation") to permanently prevent you from getting pregnant. There is also an operation for men (called a "vasectomy") to permanently prevent him from becoming pregnant.

3.5 Return of monthly bleeding

Your next normal monthly bleeding should start about 4 to 6 weeks after the abortion. The first monthly bleeding after a pill abortion may be a little heavier, or you may have more cramping or more small clots than usual.

Because you can get pregnant soon after a miscarriage, before your period returns, if you want to avoid pregnancy, start using birth control right away.

3.6 When is it safe to resume sex?

Wait at least 5 days after the abortion and 2 days after the bleeding has stopped before having sex or inserting anything into the vagina. Since the cervix was opened for the abortion, there is a greater chance of infection.

You can get pregnant a few days after the abortion. If you want to avoid pregnancy, start using a birth control method right away.

3.7 Danger signs and what to do

Seek medical attention quickly for any of these dangerous symptoms:

Heavy vaginal bleeding (soaking more than 2 pads in 1 hour for 2 hours)

Fever over 38C (100.4F)

Fever with chills or abdominal pain

Severe pain in the abdomen

Foul-smelling discharge from the vagina

Chapter 4:
Heavy Bleeding

Heavy bleeding (bleeding) after a miscarriage is a dangerous symptom. Too much blood can be fatal. If bleeding is heavy, seek medical attention if you leak more than 2 pads in 1 hour, for 2 hours, or if you have bleeding with dizziness or lightheadedness. The passage of large blood clots that are larger than an orange is also a dangerous sign.

Heavy bleeding and large clots can be caused by an incomplete miscarriage, where pieces of the pregnancy remain in the uterus (womb). To stop the bleeding, the pieces must be removed, often with abortive suction. An incomplete abortion can cause a dangerous infection.

A slow, steady trickle of bright red blood is also a danger sign. It can be caused by an injury inside you that causes you to lose too much blood.

What to do:

Get medical help immediately if you experience any of these symptoms. You will need antibiotics to prevent infection and your uterus may need to be emptied by suction. You will need someone to help you and watch for signs of shock from excessive blood loss.

4.1 Symptoms of infection: fever, abdominal pain, foul-smelling discharge

Infection after an abortion is rare but can be life-threatening. If you have any of these symptoms, seek care at a hospital or health center immediately. It means your life is in danger!

Fever:

fever with chills or severe abdominal pain

fever is over 38.5C (101.4F) and lasts for more than 4 hours

fever over 100.4°F (38°C) after a suction abortion or D&E abortion

after pill abortion fever is 38C (100.4F) and lasts more than 24 hours

Pain: severe abdominal pain

Foul-smelling discharge from the vagina

If possible, treat the infection by starting antibiotics. An untreated infection can spread to the blood (sepsis). Sepsis is very dangerous and can cause shock. Sepsis is more likely if the abortion occurred after 12 weeks of pregnancy or if the uterus (womb) was injured during the abortion.

4.2 Signs of shock

Shock is a life-threatening condition that can result from heavy bleeding. Bleeding inside the body and infection of the blood (sepsis) can also cause shock.

4.3 Danger signs:

Very fast heartbeat, more than 100 beats per minute

Pale, cold, clammy skin

Pale inner eyelids, mouth and palms

Rapid breathing, more than 30 breaths per minute

Confusion or unconsciousness (fainting)

4.4 What to do:

Get Help! Ask someone to take you to the hospital immediately!

If they are conscious

While transporting:

Lay the person down with feet higher than their head.

Keep them warm with a blanket or more clothes.

If they can drink, give sips of water or rehydration drink.

If they cannot drink, start a fast IV drip with a wide needle if you know how, or give rectal fluids.

Help them stay calm.

If they are unconscious

Lay them on their side, head low and tilted back to the side, feet higher than the head.

If they are choking, pull the tongue forward with your finger.

If they vomit, clean out the mouth immediately. Keep the head low and tilted back to the side, so no vomit is breathed into the lungs.

Do not give anything by mouth (no liquids or medicines) until the person is awake for one hour.

If you know how, start a fast IV drip with a wide needle, or start rectal fluids.

Chapter 5:

Medicines to treat infection

Tell your provider if you have ever had an allergic reaction to an antibiotic medicine. Take one of these combinations of medicines until signs of infection have been gone for 48 hours:

Combination 1:

Ceftriaxone: inject 250 mg into muscle, 1 time only;

Doxycycline: take 100 mg by mouth, 2 times a day (avoid doxycycline if you are breastfeeding);

Metronidazole: take 500 mg by mouth, 3 times a day.

Combination 2:

Ampicillin: inject 2 g (2000 mg) into muscle for the first dose only; and inject 1 g (1000 mg) for all other doses, 4 times a day;

Gentamicin: inject 80 mg into muscle, 3 times a day;

Metronidazole: take 500 mg by mouth, 3 times a day.

Combination 3:

Clindamycin: give 900 mg of intravenously (IV), 3 times a day;

Gentamicin: inject 80 mg into muscle, 3 times a day.

When the signs of infection have been gone for 48 hours: Stop giving medicines by injection or IV. Then start using both these 2 medicines by mouth with plenty of water.

Combination after signs disappear:

Doxycycline: take 100 mg by mouth, 2 times a day for 10 days (avoid taking doxycycline if you are breastfeeding); AND

Metronidazole: take 500 mg by mouth, 3 times a day for 10 days.

5.1 Estimate how many weeks pregnant you are

To know what method or methods of abortion will be best for you, you need to know how many weeks pregnant you are.

Pregnancy Calculator

Calculating gestational age at home usually involves determining the gestational age, which is the time from the first day of the last menstrual period (LMP). This is how you can estimate the age of pregnancy at home:

1. Determine the first day of your last menstrual period (LMP): This is the starting point for calculating your gestational age. Remember the date your last period started.

2. Count the weeks: Start counting the weeks from the first day of your LMP. Each week starts on the same day of the week as your LMP. For example, if your LMP was on a Monday, each subsequent week would also start on a Monday.

3. Count the days: After counting the weeks, determine the number of days that have passed since the start of your last period. For example, if you are in your seventh week and four days have passed since the beginning of this week, your total gestational age will be 7 weeks and 4 days.

4. Use a pregnancy calculator or app: If you prefer a more automated method, you can use online pregnancy calculators or smartphone apps specifically designed to estimate gestational age. These tools usually ask for the first day of your LMP and give you an estimated due date and gestational age in weeks and days.

It is important to note that this method provides an estimate and is not as accurate as medical methods such as ultrasound. A healthcare provider can use ultrasound measurements to determine gestational age with greater accuracy.

If you want a more accurate assessment of the age of your pregnancy or if you have irregular menstrual cycles or are unsure of your LMP date, it is best to consult a healthcare professional. They can perform an ultrasound scan to give you a more accurate estimate of your gestational age and due date.

 If you are more than 20 weeks pregnant, it can become more difficult to get a safe abortion.

As quickly as you can, speak with a medical professional about your options to get a safe abortion.

Aren't sure of the date for your last monthly bleeding?

If you do not remember the exact date, make the best guess you can. Try to think about events, holidays, or anything unusual that happened around the time of your monthly bleeding (for example, birthdays and other celebrations, public or school or religious holidays, sports or music events, market days, or someone coming to visit). Think about anything you did differently or did not do because you were having your monthly bleeding (buying sanitary pads).

5.2 Emergency Contraception

If you think you are less than 5 days pregnant, you can safely prevent the pregnancy by using either of 2 kinds of emergency contraception: an IUD or Emergency pills.

An IUD (Internal Uterine Device) is a birth control method that a trained health worker places in your cervix. If you get this within 5 days of unprotected sex, it will prevent pregnancy.

Emergency pills contain the same hormones as birth control pills but in different amounts. Read the instructions carefully: depending on the brand, you take 1 or 2 Emergency pills one time only; or 2 right away and another 2 pills after 12 hours. Regular birth control pills can sometimes be used as Emergency pills, but the number of pills to use and how often to take them depends on their ingredients.

Emergency pills only work in the first 5 days after unprotected sex. The earlier they are taken, the more effective they will be in preventing pregnancy.

 Headaches, nausea and abdominal pain are common side effects of emergency pills, but these should subside in a day or two. It is often normal to have light bleeding or a change in the timing of your next period.

How to take special Emergency Contraception pills
Emergency pills containing 1.5 mg (1500 mcg) levonorgestrel (*Norlevo 1.5, Plan B One-Step, Postinor-1*) Take one pill, one time only
Emergency pills containing 30 mg ulipristal acetate (*ella, ella One*) Take one pill, one time only
Emergency pills containing 0.75 mg (750 mcg) levonorgestrel (*Norlevo 0.75, Optinor, Postinor, Postinor-2, Plan B*) Take 2 pills, one time only
Emergency pills containing 50 mcg ethinyl estradiol and 250 mcg levonorgestrel (*Tetragynon*) Take 2 pills; 12 hours later, take 2 more pills.

How to take combination birth control pills for Emergency Contraception
Combined pills containing 50 mcg ethinyl estradiol and 250 mcg levonorgestrel (*Neogynon, Nordiol*) or 500 mcg norgestrel (*Ovral*) Take 2 pills; 12 hours later, take 2 more pills.
Combined pills containing 30 mcg ethinyl estradiol and 150 mcg levonorgestrel (*Microgynon, Nordette*) or 300 mcg norgestrel (*Lo-Femenal, Lo/Ovral*) Take 4 pills; 12 hours later, take 4 more pills.
Combined pills containing 20 mcg ethinyl estradiol and 100 mcg levonorgestrel (*Alesse, Lutera*) Take 5 pills; 12 hours later, take 5 more pills.

How to take mini pill birth control pills for Emergency Contraception
Progestin-only pills (minipills) containing 75 mcg norgestrel (*Ovrette*) Take 40 pills one time only
Progestin-only pills (minipills) containing 37.5 mcg levonorgestrel (*Neogest*)

Take 40 pills one time only
Progestin-only pills (minipills) containing 30 mcg levonorgestrel (*Microlut, Microval*) Take 50 pills one time only

With a pack of 21 pills, use any of the pills for Emergency contraception.

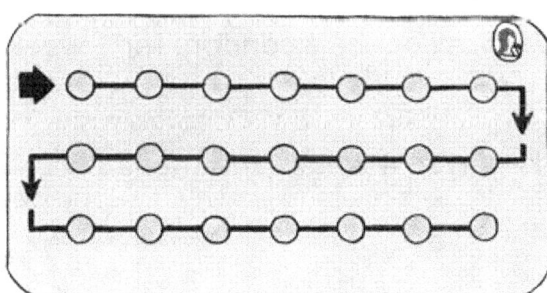

With a pack of 28 pills, use any of the first 21 pills for emergency contraception. Do not use the last 7 pills in a 28-day pack, because these pills do not contain any hormones and will not work.

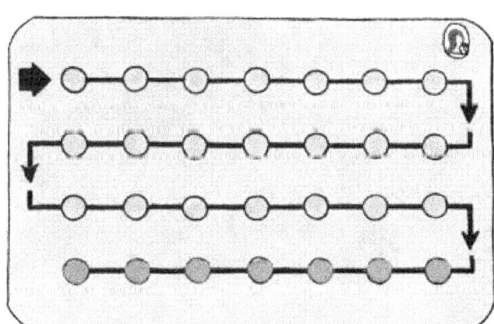

Progestin-only pills and special Emergency pills have fewer side effects (headaches and nausea) than combined pills when used for emergency contraception.

Progestin-only pills and special Emergency pills have fewer side effects (less headaches and nausea) than combined pills when used for emergency contraception.

If you are very heavy or obese, consider using the Emergency pills that contain ulipristal, or consider taking a double dose of the pills containing levonorgestrel.

If you use the Emergency pills that contain ulipristal, wait 5 days before starting hormonal methods of birth control and avoid sex or use a condom for 2 weeks to give them time to start working. It you use any of the other Emergency pills, you can start hormonal methods right away, but avoid sex or use a condom for 1 week to give them time to start working.

If you want to be sure the emergency pills worked, wait 4 weeks and then take a pregnancy test.

5.3 How to give rectal fluids

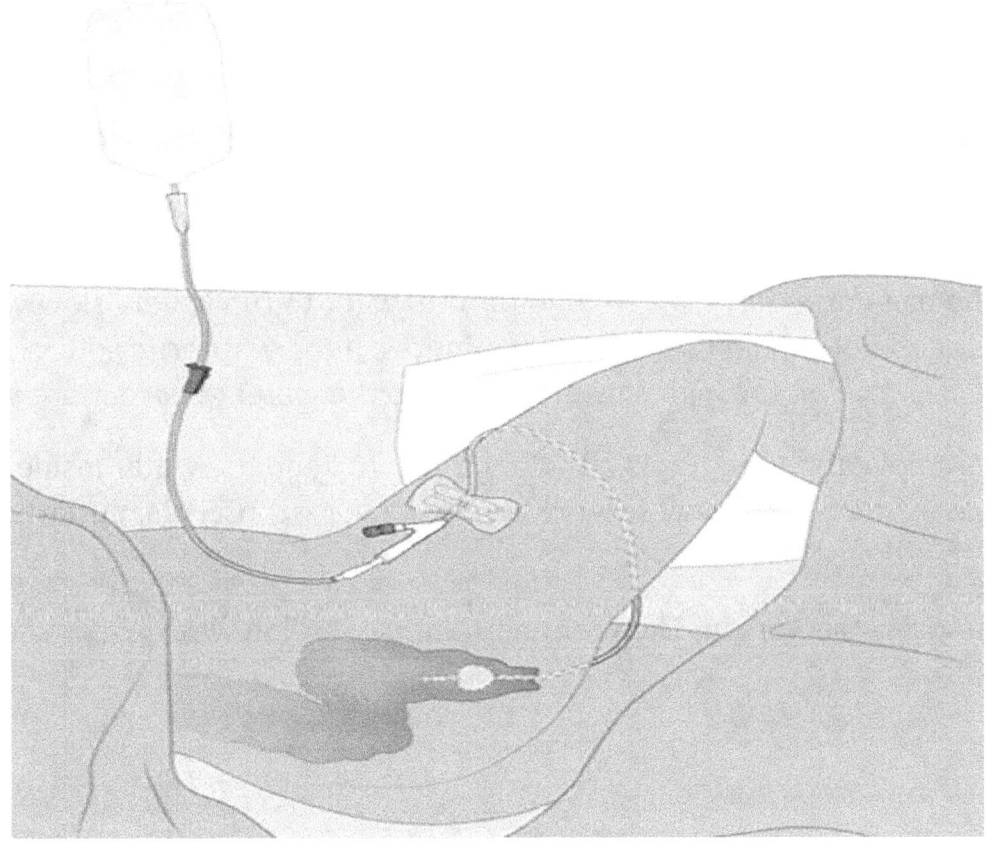

You will need:

- A clean enema bag, or a can or tin with plastic tubing.
- A cloth to place under the body.
- 600 ml (a little more than ½ a liter bottle) of warm (not hot) drinking water. Salt and sugar rehydration drink or a bag of IV solution can be used instead.

What to do:

1. Explain that because they are in serious need of fluids but cannot drink or keep them down, you are going to give fluids in the rectum, where the body will be able to absorb them.

2. Wash your hands.

3. Lying on the left side is best. To be more comfortable, put a pillow or cloth under the head.

4. If you have them, put on clean gloves.

5. Let the water come down to the end of the tube to get the air out. Then pinch the tubing to stop the flow.

6. Wet the end of the tube with water, Vaseline, or vegetable oil, and slide it into the anus. Explain that taking slow, deep breaths will help the body relax. Do not put the tube in more than 10 cm (4 inches).

7. Hold the bag or can just high enough for the water to run in very slowly. About hip level is good. It should take about 20 minutes. If the water runs out of the body, the bag may be too high. Lower the bag so the water goes in more slowly.

8. Gently remove the tube. Explain that by trying to keep the water inside, the urge to pass stool will go away soon. If the person is unconscious, push the buttocks together with your hands.

9. Clean and dry the person. Then remove your gloves and wash your hands.

Chapter 6:

Compare Methods of Abortion

While the 3 abortion methods in this book are all safe, there are differences among them that might make one method a better choice for you and your situation.

- <u>How long it takes</u>
  Pills: When misoprostol is used by itself, the abortion usually takes 7 to 8 hours, but may last up to 24 hours. If Mifepristone is taken, then 24 to 48 hours later, you take the misoprostol, the heavy bleeding and cramps will usually end 4 to 6 hours later.

Suction: A health worker uses suction in your vagina and uterus to remove the pregnancy. It takes about 10 minutes.

D&E: First the cervix is dilated (opened). If you are close to 12 weeks pregnant, this takes a few hours. If you are closer to 20 weeks, it takes longer. You will start in the clinic, go home for 1 or 2 days, and then return to the clinic. After the cervix has opened, the procedure in the clinic takes about 20 minutes.

- Pain
Pills and Suction: Both will cause mild to strong cramps off and on during the abortion. Discomfort can be lessened by taking pain medicines.

D&E: Because there can be more pain and discomfort during the abortion, you will be given lidocaine to lessen pain in the cervix and probably a strong IV pain medicine for the abortion. Cramping should stop ½ hour after the abortion.

- Bleeding
Pills: Heavy bleeding with clots is common when your body expels the pregnancy. After that, lighter bleeding may continue off and on until your monthly bleeding.

Suction: Light bleeding usually lasts one to two weeks.

D&E: There is some bleeding with small clots immediately after the abortion, then light bleeding for a few days.

- Cost
Pills and Suction: Costs vary in different countries. In the US, they cost about the same.

D&E: In the US, a D&E abortion usually costs about 1.5 to 2 times more than a suction or medical abortion.

- How often does it fail?
Pills—misoprostol only: Works 85% of the time.

Pills—misoprostol and mifepristone: Works 99% of the time.

Suction and D&E: Both work around 99% of the time.

If the pills fail, you will need a suction abortion. If a suction abortion or D&E fails, you will need to repeat it.

- <u>Advantages of each method</u>
  Pills: No antibiotics, anesthesia, instruments or tools are used. The abortion may feel more natural, like a miscarriage. It can be done as soon as you know you are pregnant. Before 10 weeks, you can do the abortion at home. You can choose to have someone with you, or you can be alone.

  Suction: The abortion is over in about 10 minutes. There is less bleeding. Health workers are with you.

  D&E: The only method recommended for use after 14 weeks. There is less
  bleeding. Health workers are with you.

- <u>Disadvantages of each method</u>
  Pills: It takes one to two days to complete the abortion. Bleeding and cramps can be heavy and can last longer than with suction or D&E.

  Suction: Instruments are put through the vagina into the uterus so the chance of infection is greater. Antibiotics or anesthetics may cause side effects. You cannot do the abortion yourself. You may not be allowed to have someone with you for support. The noise of the suction machine may be disturbing.

  D&E: It can take several hours or more than a day to complete the abortion, so you may have to go home and then return to the clinic. Strong pain medicines are often used and you may be put to sleep. Instruments are put through the vagina into the uterus, so the chance of infection is greater. Antibiotics and anesthetics may cause side effects. You cannot do the abortion yourself. You may not be allowed to have someone with you for support.

Chapter 7:

Frequently asked questions

In every country in the world, people — young and old, married and unmarried, with and without children — have abortions. One of every four pregnancies ends in abortion.

A safe abortion is just that – safe. Fewer than 1 of every 100 safe abortions lead to problems afterwards. Abortion is dangerous where it is restricted and people are denied safe abortions.

Pregnancy and birth are 10 times more dangerous than a safe abortion.

General info about abortion

- **I think I am pregnant. Can I get an abortion now?**
  If you think you may have gotten pregnant in the past 5 days, you can prevent pregnancy by using emergency contraception.

  If it has been 5 weeks or less since the first day of your last monthly bleeding, you will need a pregnancy test to find out for certain if you are pregnant. If it has been 5 or more weeks since your last period, use the pregnancy calculator to find out how far along your pregnancy is and what your abortion options are. Two thirds of abortions happen before or during the eighth week of pregnancy. While abortions are very safe, the earliest abortions are the safest.

- **How many weeks pregnant can I be and still get an abortion?**
  If the methods are available, you can get a safe abortion until you are 24 weeks pregnant. But the further along you are, the more complicated the abortion is.

  Read the chapter on **"Safe methods of abortion"**

- **Is there a minimum age to get an abortion?**
  No. Abortion with pills, suction abortions, and D&E abortions are all safe and effective methods for a person of any age.

- **Can I take abortion pills at home or do I have to go to a clinic?**
  As long as you have a way to get to a clinic quickly if a problem develops, it is safe to take abortion pills at home if you are pregnant up to 10 weeks. For pregnancies over 10 weeks, abortions with pills should be done in a clinic because help is available if you need it.

- **I have health problems. Is it safe for me to have an abortion?**
  Abortion is safe for everyone, including people with diabetes, high blood pressure, mild anemia, and other common problems. If you have severe anemia, bleeding or clotting problems, it is best to have your abortion in a clinic where help is available if needed. An abortion with pills is a better choice than a suction or D&E abortion for people who are very heavy or obese.

- **I am HIV-positive. Is it safe for me to have an abortion?**
  An abortion is just as safe for a person with HIV as for anyone else. Hopefully, you are taking anti-retrovirals (ARVs) every day to control your HIV. These medicines can keep your body strong enough to easily recover from the abortion, to make the procedure safer for your provider, and to minimize any risk of interactions with the abortion medications. If you are having an abortion at a clinic, be sure to let your provider know you are HIV-positive.

- **Where can I get pills for an abortion?**
  If abortion is legal for you, go to a women's clinic or a midwife or an ob-gyn doctor (obstetrician-gynecologist) to get counselling on how and where to get an abortion. Try to find out before you go if the clinic, midwife, or doctor has helped others get safe abortions. Depending on the laws where you live, you may also be able to get pills for an abortion (misoprostol and mifepristone) at a pharmacy. Or you may be able to get misoprostol from a midwife. If you cannot think of where else to get pills and information, look on the website of Women on Waves [https://www.womenonwaves.org/] or send them an email: info@womenonwaves.org. Also try the website of Women Help Women. [http://www.womenhelp.org/en/blog]

- **How can I know the pills are genuine?**
  Unfortunately, criminals make fake (counterfeit or pirated) pills that will not work. Try to find pills that look real: pills that are the correct size and color, that come in proper packaging, that are made by a known pharmaceutical company, that you purchase at a reputable pharmacy. Before buying them, find pictures of the pills on the internet to see what they should look like.

- **What other medicines or herbs can cause an abortion?**
  No herbs or medicines other than misoprostol and mifepristone are known to be safe and effective for abortion. People who cannot get safe abortions try many unsafe medicines, herbs, and practices which often lead to injury or death for themselves, or problems with the pregnancy if they do not succeed in causing an abortion.

- **How many times can I get an abortion before it is harmful to me?**

There is no limit to the number of abortions you can get and still be healthy. However, it is much safer and healthier to use a regular and effective birth control method.

Chapter 8:

Concerns about abortion

- <u>Will abortion affect any pregnancies I may have in the future?</u>
  Safe abortions cause no problems for future pregnancies, not for you nor any children you may have later.

- <u>Do abortions cause cancer?</u>
  Safe abortions do not cause cancer or any other illness.

- <u>Can other people (my partner, my parents) tell that I've had an abortion?</u>
  The bleeding and cramping after any kind of abortion are very similar to a very heavy period or a miscarriage. It is difficult even for a doctor to know the difference between an abortion with pills and a miscarriage.

However, if misoprostol is used vaginally, pieces of the pills may remain undissolved in the vagina for a few hours. If this could cause a problem for you, it is better to take misoprostol by mouth.

- **How can I find out about the laws regarding abortion where I live?**
  Laws regarding abortion are different from country to country, and often vary in different parts of the same country. Until abortion is safe and legal everywhere, you can use the Center for Reproductive Rights [http://worldabortionlaws.com/] website to find out about the laws concerning abortions all around the world.

- **How can I tell if an abortion will be safe?**
  Luckily, abortions with pills are usually very safe because nothing is put inside your uterus (womb), which is what causes infections or injuries in unsafe abortions. It is not always easy to tell if a suction abortion or D&E will be safe. You can go ask questions of the provider, or ask another person who was treated there.

  - Will they answer your questions? They should if they have nothing to hide.
  - Has anyone gotten sick or died from having an abortion there? If so, go somewhere else.
  - Who will do the abortion? How and where were they trained? Doctors, nurses, and other health workers can do safe abortions if they have been trained in safe abortion methods and infection prevention.
  - Does the clinic seem to be clean and neat? If it is dirty and messy, the abortion might be that way too.
  - Is there a place for washing hands where they do the abortions? If a health worker cannot wash hands, there can be no safe abortion.
  - How do they clean their instruments and tools? All tools and instruments should be sterilized.
  - Does the cost seem fair? If the cost is very high, it may mean the health worker cares more about your money than your health.
  - Do they also provide services like family planning, treatment of STIs or HIV, and counselling? A good clinic cares about your entire reproductive health.

o What will they do if something goes wrong? Every clinic should have a plan to get you to a hospital in case of emergency.

After visiting an abortion provider, if you have doubts about whether an abortion there will be safe, trust your feelings and leave. Look for another clinic that feels safer.

Chapter 9:

Preparing for an abortion

Preparing for an abortion is an important step in ensuring a smooth and comfortable experience. This chapter provides a comprehensive guide to the necessary preparations, including securing support, gathering essential supplies, preparing for emergencies, and managing potential side effects. By being well prepared, you can go through the abortion process with more confidence and peace of mind.

9.1 What kind of help will I need?

Having someone to support you throughout the abortion process is essential, especially if unforeseen complications arise. Consider having a friend or family member accompany you to support you, whether you choose to have an abortion at the clinic or take the medication at home. Their presence can provide emotional support and help with logistical matters such as transportation to and from the clinic or hospital.

9.2 What aids should I have during and after a pill abortion?

To ensure your comfort and well-being during and after a medical abortion, it is important to have the following items on hand:

9.2.1 Menstrual pads:

Have an adequate supply of menstrual pads to manage the bleeding that occurs during and after the abortion. It is advisable to choose pads instead of tampons to reduce the risk of infection.

9.2.2 Mild soap:

Keep a mild, unscented soap on hand to maintain personal hygiene during the abortion process. Use soap to gently clean the external genitalia.

9.2.3 Painkillers:

You may experience cramping and discomfort during the abortion process. It may be helpful to have pain relievers such as aspirin or ibuprofen available to relieve pain. However, consult your healthcare provider before taking any medication to ensure its safety and suitability for your particular situation.

9.2.4 Antibiotics:

Although the risk of infection after a miscarriage is low, it is wise to be prepared. Talk to your healthcare provider ahead of time and ask if antibiotics are necessary as a precaution. If infection occurs, early treatment with antibiotics may be essential.

9.2.5 Heating pad or hot water bottle:

Cramps are a common side effect of abortion. Having a heating pad or hot water bottle can provide relief and help soothe abdominal discomfort. Apply heat to the lower abdomen for a short time, making sure the temperature is comfortable to avoid burns.

9.2.6 Hydration and snacks:

Staying hydrated is essential during the abortion process. Have plenty of water available to drink and rehydrate. Additionally, keep some light snacks on hand to stave off hunger and provide nutrition. Opt for easily digestible foods that do not cause nausea.

9.3 Emergency preparedness:

Although it is rare, it is important to be prepared for emergency situations. Consider the following:

9.3.1 Emergency contacts:

Make sure you identify a reliable person who can take you to a hospital or clinic in an emergency. Share their contact information with trusted individuals who can help in an emergency.

9.3.2 Hospital or clinic address:

Write down the exact address of the hospital or clinic where you would prefer medical help in an emergency. Having this information readily available will speed up the process when needed.

9.4 What can I do to make me feel less sick from abortion drugs?

Nausea is a potential side effect of abortion medications, but there are steps you can take to minimize discomfort. Consider the following tips:

9.4.1 Eat small meals:

Eat a small meal before taking the abortion pill. Avoid overeating as a full stomach can make nausea worse.

9.4.2 Stay hydrated:

Drink plenty of water during the abortion process to prevent dehydration, which can increase feelings of nausea. Maintaining adequate hydration is important for your overall well-being.

9.4.3 Consider nausea-relieving foods and drinks:

Certain foods and drinks can help ease nausea during the abortion process. Try including the following in your diet:

- Apple slices: Apples contain fiber, which helps with digestion and reduces nausea.

- Bananas: Rich in potassium, bananas can help balance electrolytes and ease nausea.

- Cookies: Eating plain cookies can help absorb stomach acid and provide a mild, soothing effect on the stomach.

- Broth, ginger or mint tea: Sipping warm broth or herbal teas made with ginger or mint can soothe the stomach and ease nausea.

- Aromatherapy: Consider using aromatherapy techniques by inhaling the scents of ginger, mint, or lemon, as these scents are known to have a calming effect on some individuals.

- Muscle relaxation techniques: Some people find relief from nausea by stretching their back and neck muscles. Gentle stretching exercises or relaxation techniques can help relieve discomfort.

9.4.4 Acupressure:

Applying pressure to specific points on the body, such as the P6 point located above the inner wrist, can help relieve nausea. This technique, known as acupressure, can be done on your own or by a trained practitioner.

Conclusion:

Chapter 9 provided valuable insights on how to prepare for an abortion. By having a support system, gathering essential supplies, preparing for emergencies, and managing potential side effects like nausea, you can approach the abortion process with more confidence and comfort. Be sure to consult with healthcare professionals for individualized advice and recommendations based on your specific circumstances. Preparation is key to ensuring a smooth and safe abortion, and by taking the necessary steps outlined in this chapter, you can navigate the process more easily.

Chapter 10:

After an abortion

After you've had an abortion, it's important to understand what to expect during the recovery process and how to ensure your health moving forward. This chapter provides comprehensive information on the symptoms that indicate a successful abortion procedure and offers advice on post-abortion care, emotional support, resuming physical activity and preventing future pregnancies. By being aware of what is normal and taking the necessary precautions, you can navigate the post-abortion period with confidence.

10.1 How do I know that the abortion has worked?

After an abortion, whether it was a medical abortion or a suction/surgical abortion, the signs of pregnancy gradually disappear. It is natural to be concerned about the effectiveness of the procedure. Here are some indicators that the abortion was successful:

10.1.1 Disappearance of pregnancy symptoms:

After an abortion, pregnancy symptoms such as morning sickness (nausea) and breast tenderness subside. Morning sickness usually subsides within a day, while breast tenderness subsides quickly after suctioning or surgical abortion. In the case of medical abortion, breast tenderness may persist for about a week.

10.1.2 Ultrasound confirmation:

To confirm the success of the abortion procedure, you may consider having an ultrasound (sonogram) performed at the clinic. An ultrasound can provide visual proof that the pregnancy has been terminated, giving you peace of mind.

It is important to note that the symptoms of a miscarriage, including bleeding, cramping, and pain in the lower back or abdomen, are similar to those of a miscarriage. In places where abortion is not legally available, expressing concern about a possible abortion can be a way to seek needed medical help.

10.2 Who can I talk to afterwards?

Processing your emotions and experiences after a miscarriage is an essential part of the healing process. It can be helpful to talk to others who have been through similar situations, or to find a supportive friend who can offer understanding and empathy. It's normal to experience a range of emotions after a miscarriage, including relief, sadness, grief, guilt, shame, anger, and even love. However, having to hide these feelings or pretend that nothing happened can intensify negative emotions. Look for non-judgmental support systems, such as counseling services or support groups, to help you navigate your emotional journey.

10.3 How long should I wait before engaging in strenuous activities?

The most important aspect of miscarriage recovery is to listen to your body and give it the time it needs to heal. Although there are no specific scientific guidelines, it is generally recommended to wait before resuming strenuous activities. Consider the following recommendations:

10.3.1 Less than 13 weeks of pregnancy:

If your pregnancy was terminated before the 13th week, it is recommended to wait approximately 4-7 days before engaging in sports or activities that require physical exertion.

10.3.2 More than 13 weeks of pregnancy:

For pregnancies terminated after 13 weeks, it is advisable to wait closer to 14 days before participating in strenuous activities. The recovery process may require additional time due to the advanced stage of pregnancy.

The key is to listen to your body, rest and gradually increase your physical activity as you regain strength.

10.4 How long should I wait before resuming sexual activity?

Resuming sexual activity after an abortion requires careful consideration and taking the necessary precautions. It is important to give the body time to heal and reduce the risk of complications. Here are some guidelines to follow:

10.4.1 Wait at least 5 days:

After an abortion, wait at least 5 days before engaging in intercourse. This time frame allows your body to recover and reduces the risk of infection.

10.4.2 Wait until the bleeding stops:

In addition, wait until the bleeding from the abortion has completely stopped before resuming sexual activity. This will ensure that your body fully heals and reduce the risk of infection.

10.4.3 Use of contraception:

It's important to remember that you can get pregnant again a few days after a miscarriage. If you do not wish to become pregnant, it is essential to start a reliable method of contraception. Consider discussing birth control options with your healthcare provider to determine the most appropriate method for your needs and preferences. Starting birth control before resuming sexual activity will help prevent unwanted pregnancy.

10.5 When can I get pregnant again?

After an abortion, it is possible to get pregnant shortly afterwards. If you want to avoid pregnancy, it is essential to start using a contraceptive method immediately. Contraceptive methods are highly effective in preventing pregnancy when used correctly. Consult with your healthcare provider to choose a method that fits your reproductive goals and preferences.

Conclusion:

This chapter provided valuable information regarding the post-abortion period. You now have a better understanding of how to determine if the abortion procedure was successful, the importance of seeking emotional support, the recommended waiting time before beginning strenuous activity, and what precautions to take before resuming sexual activity. Remember to prioritize your physical and emotional well-being during this period. If you have any concerns or questions, don't hesitate to contact healthcare professionals who can offer advice and support. By taking care of yourself and making informed decisions, you can navigate the post-abortion phase with confidence and move forward on your personal journey.

Chapter 11:
What can I do to prevent future pregnancy?

After you've had an abortion, it's crucial to consider your options for preventing future pregnancies. Taking control of your reproductive health allows you to plan and make decisions that align with your goals and desires. This chapter explores the different birth control methods available to you and allows you to choose the option that best suits your needs and preferences. Whether you're looking for short-term protection or a more permanent solution, understanding the different birth control methods will help you make informed decisions.

11.1 Choosing a contraceptive method:

There are many contraceptive methods to prevent future pregnancy. It is important to choose a method that fits your lifestyle, personal preferences and overall health. Here are three broad categories of birth control to consider:

11.1.1 Barrier methods:

Barrier methods create a physical barrier that prevents sperm from reaching the egg, reducing the risk of pregnancy. These methods include:

- Condoms: Male and female condoms are effective in preventing pregnancy and the transmission of sexually transmitted infections (STIs).

- Diaphragm: The diaphragm is a silicone or latex cup that covers the cervix and prevents sperm from entering the uterus.

11.1.2 Hormonal methods:

Hormonal birth control methods involve the use of synthetic hormones to prevent ovulation and alter cervical mucus, making it harder for sperm to reach the egg. These methods include:

- Birth control pills: Oral contraceptives are taken daily and contain hormones that prevent ovulation.

- Injection: Injectable contraception, administered every few months, releases hormones to inhibit ovulation.

11.1.3 Long-acting reversible methods (LARC):

Long-acting reversible contraceptive methods are highly effective and provide protection for a longer period of time without requiring daily or frequent use. LARC options include:

- Intrauterine devices (IUDs): Small T-shaped bodies inserted into the uterus to prevent pregnancy for several years.

- Implants: Small rods inserted under the skin that release hormones to prevent pregnancy for several years.

11.2 Options for permanent contraception:

If you're sure you don't want any more children, permanent birth control options are available. These methods are considered permanent because they cannot be easily undone. They contain:

- **Tubal ligation:** Also known as "tubal ligation" is a surgical procedure in which the fallopian tubes are blocked or severed, preventing the eggs from reaching the uterus.

- **Vasectomy**: A vasectomy is a male surgery that cuts or blocks the tubes that carry sperm from the testicles, resulting in permanent infertility.

It is important to note that permanent methods should be carefully considered as they are not reversible or easily reversed. Before making a decision, it may be helpful to discuss your options with a healthcare provider who can provide guidance and ensure you have all the information you need.

Conclusion:

Preventing future pregnancies is a fundamental aspect of reproductive health and family planning. In this chapter, we explored different contraceptive methods, from barrier methods to hormonal options and long-acting reversible methods. We also discussed permanent birth control options for individuals who are certain they do not want to become pregnant in the future. By understanding your options and seeking advice from healthcare professionals, you will be able to make informed decisions about your reproductive journey and take control of your reproductive health. Remember that birth control choices are personal and what works for one person may not work for another.